I0481505

To Binge Or Not To Binge

Ideas On How To Stop Binge Eating and Overeating Forever And Sticking to A Healthy Food Plan

BY

Roy Mckenzie

© Copyright 2018 by _____ - All rights reserved.

The following eBook is reproduced below with the goal of providing information that is as accurate and reliable as possible. Regardless, purchasing this eBook can be seen as consent to the fact that both the publisher and the author of this book are in no way experts on the topics discussed within and that any recommendations or suggestions that are made herein are for entertainment purposes only. Professionals should be consulted as needed, prior to undertaking any of the action endorsed herein.

This declaration is deemed fair and valid by both the American Bar Association and the Committee of Publishers Association and is legally binding throughout the United States.

Furthermore, the transmission, duplication or reproduction of any of the following work including specific information will be considered an illegal act irrespective of if it is done electronically or in print. This extends to creating a secondary or tertiary copy of the work or a recorded copy and is only allowed with an express written consent from the Publisher. All additional right reserved.

The information in the following pages is broadly considered to be a truthful and accurate account of facts, and as such any inattention, use or misuse of the information in question by the reader will render any resulting actions solely under their purview. There are no scenarios in which the publisher or the original author of this work can be in any fashion deemed liable for any hardship or damages that may befall them after undertaking information described herein.

Additionally, the information in the following pages is intended only for informational purposes and should thus be thought of as universal. As befitting its nature, it is presented without assurance regarding its prolonged validity or interim quality. Trademarks that are mentioned are done without written consent and can in no way be considered an endorsement from the trademark holder.

TABLE OF CONTENTS

INTRODUCTION

Thank you for taking the time to download this book: *To Binge or Not To Binge*

This book covers the topic of binge eating and will teach you some easy steps and ideas to stop binge eating for good.

At the completion of this book, you will have a good understanding of binge eating and be able to live a happy and healthier lifestyle.

Once again, thanks for downloading this book, I hope you find it to be helpful!

CHAPTER 1

What is Binge Eating?

Binge eating, according to the dictionary, is a "period of excessive eating" (Dictionary). These episodes of binge eating are described in a few ways; the first is, in a set time frame, for example, an hour, one consumes a certain amount of food that is obviously greater than what an average person would eat under the same circumstances. Due to varying body types and metabolisms, the amount of food one consumes on a daily basis can differ; however, with common sense, one knows if they are eating a larger portion than normal. The second description of binge eating describes it as, "a sense of lack of control over eating during the episode (e.g., a feeling that one cannot stop eating or control what or how much one is eating)" (National eating disorder). Some telltale signs that one is binge eating are: eating quicker than usual, eating till discomfort, eating despite not being hungry, eating in seclusion because one is embarrassed about how much they eat and having a guilty sensation after eating. In this case, binge eating becomes a mental issue not just a physical one.

Regardless of the problems origin—mental or physical—the main problem stems from overeating.

Often, these periods of excessive eating are associated with the common eating disorder, binge eating disorder. Binge eating disorder is a serious disease, and in severe cases, it can be life-threatening. The disease itself is "characterized by recurrent episodes of eating large quantities of food (often very quickly and to the point of discomfort)" (National eating disorder). Because of the nature of the disease, the person suffering from the disease is fully aware of the fact that they are overeating. They feel a sense of loss of control during the binge; therefore, it is not uncommon to experience emotions such as shame, guilt, and distress. These strong emotions can cause a variety of other health issues that stem from the original disorder, Binge Eating Disorder.

During a binge eating episode, numerous calories are consumed rapidly without a chance to burn them off. The shame and guilt caused by the knowledge of how those calories will affect one's image can force a person to seek out unhealthy alternatives to exercise such as, purging. Purging, or throwing up after eating, is directly linked to another disease called bulimia, and frequently these two eating disorders appear together. They do this to counter the effects of the binge eating, but bulimia has its own set of side effects other than keeping off the weight. This is a severe disease, and "is the most common eating disorder in the United States" (National eating disorder).

Although purging is the most popular form of combating binge eating, some people go one step further and will stop eating altogether; thus, we see anorexia as another way of tackling binge eating disorder. However, a person who has binge eaten can become so disgusted with themselves that their mental image of their appearance can be ruined. When this occurs, anorexia takes a severe form, and the person can refuse to eat even though they have already lost a lot of weight.

As mentioned before, binge eating is not only a physical disorder; it is a mental one as well. Because of the strong emotions like, guilt and shame that are connected to the binging episodes—usually occurring three to four times a month—people can very easily slide into depression. When depression sinks in it is essential to see a specialist.

Furthermore, binge eating is not something to be taken lightly.

Binge eating disorder does not stereotype and does not only effect a particular demographic. Although it usually starts in the early twenties, there have been many cases observed in older adults. And, according to a study conducted by the National Eating Disorder Agency (NEDA); out of roughly nine thousand "English speaking Americans" approximately forty percent of the group with binge eating disorder" were male" (National eating disorder). In people looking for a weight loss treatment with thirty percent of them "show signs" of binge eating disorder" (National eating disorder). Binge eating is considered one of the newest eating disorders, finally being classified in 2013, and it is not as well-known as some of the other eating diseases mentioned above, but it can be equally, if not more dangerous to one's health.

CHAPTER 2

Causes, Prevention, and Repercussions of Binge Eating

Researchers have yet to find the exact reason some people develop binge eating disorder, but have recognised certain things that contribute to its development. As mentioned in the previous chapter, binge eating disorder can lead to the development of other diseases such as bulimia, anorexia, and depression, what wasn't said, was that this could work as a two-way street. Like these diseases, binge eating disorder forms from a combination of psychological, biological and environmental factors.

Usually, binge eating disease stems from some previous mental health issue such as depression. "Nearly half of all people diagnosed with binge eating disorder have a history of depression" (WebMD). Of course, the link isn't visible, but people suffering from binge eating complain about emotions like frustration, sadness, monotony, and nervousness along with other pessimistic feelings bringing on a bout of binge eating. Also, it is important to note that sporadic and spontaneous decision making is common with binge eating disorder.

This is because people who act impulsively usually show a lack of self-control.

In cases like these, where the person suffering from an eating disease has previous mental issues, binge eating can stem from medications prescribed. Some drugs have an adverse side effect that prevents a person from recognizing they are full. The medicines prevent messages to the brain "that stimulate appetite and may interfere with people being able to sense" they do not need any more "food after a meal" (WebMD).

There is a widespread theory amongst specialists that binge eating—and other eating disorders—are inherited. Eating disorders tend to run in families; if one's close family member suffered from one of these diseases—bulimia, anorexia, and binge eating disorder—chances are much higher that they will contract the disease as well. "Researchers are looking into the possible abnormal functioning of chemical messages to the brain involving hormones that regulate appetite such as leptin and ghrelin (WebMD). If a correlation can be drawn, then they will be able to link an inherited aptitude for eating disorders directly. Another reason why researchers are trying to link eating disorders—and binge eating specifically—to an inherited trait is because, more often than not, binge eaters tend to come from families that overeat or "put an unnatural emphasis on food" (WebMD). Situations like this arise when food is viewed as a reward. For example, if someone were to do a good job, they would receive a steak dinner or their favorite meal. This leads to food becoming a source of comfort and happiness. Once this occurs, food is eaten as a learned response to undesirable circumstances or stress.

Unfortunately, binge eating does not have a cure. It is impossible to prevent because until one displays symptoms, it is impossible to tell that they will. However, it is crucial that one begins treatment as soon as they start to show any of the symptoms mentioned in chapter one. Also, education is essential. Learning and encouraging healthy eating habits, along with sensible stances on food and body image are also very helpful in the prevention of not only binge eating, but all sorts of other eating disorders. So far, the age-old saying, knowledge is power, still rings true when it comes to eating disorders. The more one knows, the quicker one can realize what is happening to them, and the faster they can react to prevent a negative outcome.

When the worst occurs, and one gives in to binge eating, some emotional and physical consequences arise. For example, instantly after binging one fills with "shame, self-hatred, anxiety, and depression" (Disorderhope). On the physical side of things, one feels uncomfortable from eating too much food and can feel "gastrointestinal distress" "due to the high volume of food ingested" (Disorderhope). On top of these feelings, a person may feel exhausted because their body is working so hard on digesting the large amount of food they have just consumed. These are only a few of the short-term effects of binge eating; the consequences to one's health are much more severe.

When one binge eats the body responds differently than it would when it consumes a reasonable amount of food. The massive caloric intake at once sends the body into survival mode and it will begin to store everything that it has eaten in fat cells. Although some binge eaters maintain a healthy weight, many of them gain significant amounts of weight; thus, the health risks associated with binge eating are very similar to clinical obesity. Some of these health risks are as follows: high blood pressure, high cholesterol levels, heart disease—as a result of high triglyceride levels—diabetes (type 2), and gallbladder disease (National eating disorder); however, this is not the end, many of these side-effects can transform into other problems. High blood pressure and high cholesterol place strain on the heart and can result in a heart attack. And, diabetes, if not appropriately treated, can lead to kidney and nerve damage, and in some severe cases those who suffer see the signs of early onset Alzheimer's disease. It is essential for someone who is starting to see the first symptoms of binge eating disorder that they see a doctor immediately and start treatment as soon as possible.

CHAPTER 3

Steps to Follow to Break the Habit

The previous chapter discussed how and what the treatments are for binge eating and this may be precisely the route that some people need to take to get better; however, binge eating can be a complicated problem to overcome because food is an essential part of life. In contrast to drinking and smoking, food cannot just be removed from one's everyday routine. The following steps are not a sure fire way to kick one's binge eating habits, but they may assist or help cope with binge eating disorder.

The very first thing that someone needs to do when they think that they have binge eating disorder is to tell someone. It could be a trusted friend, spouse, or a family member. Now, this may be very difficult because it is a personal and frankly embarrassing topic to talk about, but someone other than the person suffering needs to know. This is important for two reasons. One, very simply this allows the person with binge eating disorder to no longer feel alone in their struggle. They now have someone in their corner that they can talk about certain issues with rather than bottling them up inside, and quite possibly lead to a binge eating episode. The second reason that it is important to tell someone is for medical reasons. If something were to happen to the person with binge eating disorder than the medical staff that is treating them needs to know what is going on with their patient. And, if said patient is incapacitated then there needs to be someone privy to that kind of information.

Now that the cat is out of the bag, it is time to seek help from a professional. Telling the first person is the hardest. It is admitting to yourself, as well as one other person that you have a problem. After that, enrolling in an eating disorder treatment facility or signing up for therapy sessions should be much more agreeable. As uncomfortable as these first two steps are, one needs to be willing to accept help and learn how to make themselves vulnerable, or else they could never get better.

Now that the hard part is over it is time to relax. Telling someone you have a problem and enrolling in an eating disorder treatment facility are difficult things to do. Once one has done that, they can take solace in the fact that they have made steps towards their recovery. Perhaps, it would be an excellent time to set some time aside to enjoy life and be happy before the treatment begins. Find a fun, physically active pursuit and go out and participate.

After one relaxes a little bit and comes to grips with the eating disorder, it is time to forgive oneself. There is no point in toiling over past episodes because there is nothing that can be done to change it. Therefore, these mistakes should no longer represent failure; they should act as pillars of knowledge. One should go back, and remember what their mother told them all those years ago when they did something wrong, "learn from your mistakes."

At this point, it is time to take action and speak to a nutritionist. Not only will these people advise what to avoid as far as fatty foods, but they will help to set up a healthy meal plan to ensure that all the necessary vitamins are still being consumed without overeating. Once one has visited and discussed what they need from the nutritionist, it is smart to take this information and put it to work by constructing a strict meal plan each week; an idea that will not be deviated from at all.

Because you have taken the time to set up a meal plan and visit a nutritionist, there is no need to start dieting. These fad diets rarely help for an extended period and if anything they make one more susceptible to relapse. Restriction places certain foods on a pedestal and makes them appear more desirable. One always wants what they cannot have.

After creating a meal plan with a nutritionist, one should only have the necessary food in the house; however one can still have a binge eating episode. An excellent way to prevent relapse is to limit what food is lying around the house. Granted, this may become a little bit of a hassle, but it would be a good idea to do the grocery shopping each day. Once one has consulted their meal plan, they could go to the grocery store and only buy what they need for the day. That way there will be an insufficient amount of temptation around the house, and one would have to physically leave their home to binge eat.

Another way to prevent binge eating is making sure that one eats breakfast every day. It sounds strange—eating food to avoid eating food—but it works. In North American society breakfast has all but been done away with. Because people are waking up earlier and going to work earlier it gets forgotten about, and then those that skip it end up eating larger portions later on in the day. If one eats breakfast, their stomach is much more settled, and they do not need to eat a huge meal at lunchtime to make up for it; thus, preventing a possible binge eating episode.

Other than making sure one eats regular meals, it is essential to make sure that one gets all of the vitamins and nutrients that the body needs. Of course, a nutritionist will ensure that any meal plan one makes with them will include all of the essential things one needs to stay healthy, but just in case, it is a good idea to take multi-vitamins and mineral supplements. Like breakfast, other meals can sometimes be skipped. In situations like this, it is smart to have a backup plan such as said multi-vitamins and mineral supplements. This way one can ensure—despite forgetting meals—they are staying as healthy as possible.

Eating healthy and making sure the body gets everything that it needs is not the only things one can do to stay healthy. Exercise is critical especially for those suffering from binge eating disorder. Binge eating often leads to weight gain and subsequently a terrible personal image. As mentioned before, half of the battle against binge eating disorder is dealing with the side effects of weight gain. Having a planned regiment that one is willing to maintain can help battle the dreaded weight gain that is paired with binge eating; however, if the regiment is not able to be kept then it can have the reverse effect. It can make one think that they cannot accomplish something as fundamental as a workout routine. That being said, exercise just feels right. It sends endorphins through the bloodstream and makes one feel good about themselves which can be especially helpful if they are dealing with image issues or a disorder like binge eating.

Everything mentioned above are practical steps towards getting help with binge eating disorder. From here on out, the rest of these steps are additional things that someone can do to get well, and many of them will most likely be recommended by one's therapist.

For starters, in therapy one should determine their binge eating trigger. Once these causes and triggers of binge eating have been illuminated, it is on the shoulders of the one who is suffering from binge eating to avoid them at all costs. Talking about them can only do so much. One needs to change their lifestyle, friendship circle, or hobbies whatever it takes to avoid these triggers because all they will do is lead one directly back into binge eating. By establishing these things and making a plan to prevent them, one is taking steps in preventing further binge eating episodes.

To help assist in avoiding these causes and triggers of binge eating, joining a self-help group is a good idea. This allows one to voice their opinions and feelings about giving up said people and activities that lead to binge eating. Doing it oneself is extremely difficult, and a support group will allow one to vent and continue to maintain their new lifestyle. Not only will it provide one with a place to vent about their troubles, but it will also show them that they are not alone in the battle against binge eating disorder.

On top of joining a support group and giving oneself a group to which they can voice their feelings, it is important to include one's current friendship group. Regardless of the fact that it might be embarrassing to tell one's friends that they are suffering, or if they are a source of the binge eating episodes, the only way that they can help is if they know what is going on. Furthermore, if they are a source of your binge eating episodes, they need to know your concerns. This way, they may be able to alter the way they act or what they say around who are suffering. Not to mention, it is important to never isolate oneself from anyone that can help the situation.

On the other side of things, there are plenty of things that can be done without other people to help improve one's binge eating disorder. To begin with, finding a good self-help book will teach excellent practices for improving one's life. They will also give helpful advice in dealing with your disorder, primarily if it the book is centered on binge eating disorder.

Another good thing to do is starting writing in a journal. Journals help keep track of emotions and reactions to said emotions. Writing all of the feelings down will help one to recognize when an episode could be coming. It could help identify specific causes and triggers; and, learn how to avoid them. Also, writing things down can help get things off of their chest, rather than resorting to binge eating. This is much healthier than ending up eating an entire pantry full of cookies.

Finally, and as cliché, as it sounds, the last is not the least important. The best step one can take towards recovering from binge eating disorder—or any disease for that matter—is love themselves. Loving oneself, rather than what one looks like allows for the smaller victories to be celebrated. Looking at oneself in a negative light will never permit them to get healthy. The image is not the most important thing and recognizing that will go a long way in the fight against binge eating disorder.

Long story short, binge eating disorder often requires the assistance of a support group, therapist, or a treatment center. If one is fighting binge eating and would like to seek improvement, they should call one of the residential centers today and not wait for things to get worse. These treatment centers provide an excellent assortment of treatment options, excellent staffs, and a variety of therapy types. In conclusion, these treatment centers have been proven exceptionally beneficial in treating binge eating disorder and preventing relapse.

CHAPTER 4

Self-Help, Clinical, and Holistic Treatments for Binge Eating

Like any disorder, the first step to improving is to admit to the problem. One must resign their pride and accept the fact that they are sick; binge eating disorder is no different. Once the problem has been illuminated there are some avenues one can take towards getting better, and a lot of them are through self-help. That being said, because of the nature of binge eating disorder, and its ability to affect one physically and mentally, it is crucial to involve a professional to ensure the prevention of a relapse. And, if one chooses to go this route, there are now federal drug administration approved drugs out there specifically designed to combat binge eating disorder. The critical thing to remember is that there are many avenues which one can get healthy and return to healthy eating habits, and no way is the wrong way.

When people think of self-help, they believe that it is alone; however, that is far from the truth. After admitting the problem—

binge eating—a person should see a doctor and explain to them the issue. Usually, the preliminary step—if the problem isn't severe—will be a guided self-help book. The book itself contains many good practices that will help the reader develop good habits to combat binge eating, but act of self-help—guided or not—is a form of treatment; Although you will have regular meetings with a physician, it helps rebuild the readers confidence in themselves; it helps them believe that they can beat binge eating disorder.

As one works through this book—alongside their doctor—they will illuminate different practices that will directly influence their binge eating. For example, one method could be setting out a structured meal plan. Each week, one would—in detail—write out every meal for each day. Creating a plan for your eating will help you regulate what you take into your body; thus, you will prevent hunger but also avoid binge eating. Anything that isn't on your list is not allowed to be consumed. Additionally, the plan makes the creator privy to an easy to read list of what they are putting into their body. This will help you notice what healthy and unhealthy foods you are putting into your body and— with help from a professional—identify patterns in your behavior. Another important thing that these books will help one understand is their triggers, what exactly sends them into a binge eating frenzy. If one can identify what it is that makes them want to binge eat; perhaps they will be able to walk away from the said trigger and prevent a binge eating episode. Once the triggers have been discovered, it will be easier to find out what the underlying causes are of your binge eating, allowing you to work through these issues in a smart and healthier way. If you are being sent on an eating binge, these emotions are strong, and it is essential to find a better way to manage them, and your weight in an intelligent manner. While working through the self-help book, some people may start to feel very alone, despite regular discussions with their physician. The right way to resist these lonely feelings, which could put you at risk of a binge eating episode, is to join a self-help group. It doesn't need to be Alcoholics Anonymous, who will undoubtedly allow you to join—they talk about more than just alcohol—it can be something online. One group, called BEAT is a specific support group that focuses on binge eating. Support is essential when battling against any disease and binge eating is no different.

Self-help is a popular way to fight against binge eating disorder, but at times it isn't enough just by itself. Usually, a doctor will allow you a four-week trial period to see if there are improvements. If there hasn't been sufficient steps taken towards recovery, the next step is to begin cognitive behavior therapy (NHS).

If one has been offered cognitive behavior therapy, it can come in two ways. Usually, it will "be in group sessions with other people"; however, there are some instances that they will offer private sessions with a therapist (NHS). Cognitive behavior therapy runs for about four months, with there being one meeting each week—sixteen sessions total. The group sessions are longer because there is less personal interaction with the therapist. They usually run for ninety minutes, and the private sessions will go for an hour.

Cognitive behavior therapy "involves talking with a therapist, who will help you explore patterns of thoughts, feelings, and behaviors that could be contributing to your eating disorder" (NHS). As mentioned before, binge eating disorder is as much mental as it is physical, and it is essential to discover precisely what it is that is contributing to the need to binge eat.

Similar to the self-help regiment, cognitive behavior therapy will help you set out a plan for your eating habits. They will assist one in constructing a healthy plan for meals and snacks that will assist in abolishing the harmful eating habits and creating regular ones. Triggers will also be addressed. The triggers one addressed during their self-help stage will be discussed once again, but the therapist will look at your triggers with a much more critical eye. Hopefully, they will find some that had not been discovered yet; thus, providing a possible explanation as to why the self-help stage was not entirely successful. Also, one's feelings and emotions will be talked about. The therapist will attempt to "change and manage" negative feelings about one's body (NHS). These feelings tend to be what leads to an episode, and they need to be kept in check. Finally, cognitive behavior therapy will strive to keep one on track. The new eating habits formed in the self-help part and the therapy sections of one's rehabilitation are only helpful if they are sustained. The group setting will aid as a support group to help one overcome their disease.

As one can see, many of the same practices are performed in cognitive behavior therapy as are performed in the self-help portion of treatment. What sets therapy apart from self-help is the feelings of not being alone. The online support groups are good, but at times one needs reassurance in person. The group therapy sessions—and even the private sessions—provide one with an actual face to share problems with as well as meeting with other people suffering from the same thing that you are, and tells you that you are not alone in the fight. Therapy is one of the best ways to deal with binge eating disorder, but its track record is not perfect; if the sessions fail to provide sufficient results, the final treatment for binge eating disorder is medication.

Medication is the last line of defense against binge eating because physicians try to remedy the problem with natural ways before unnatural ones. Doctors tend to have two ways of medicating a patient suffering from binge eating disorder; one, they try to use physiological drugs to stop the episodes preemptively. And two, they attempt to medicate the cause or the result of your binge eating disorder (e.g., depression). Although these medications have had great success with combating binge eating disorder, they only affect a specific aspect of the disease—they cannot prevent or stop the disorder entirely without the added assistance that therapy and self-help books provide.

After self-help and cognitive behavior therapy has failed to provide sufficient results, the first medication that doctors often prescribe Lisdexamfetamine (Vyvanse). Lisdexamfetamine "is approved by the FDA to treat binge eating disorder" (WebMD). If this name seems familiar, it is because this drug is also used to treat ADHD; however, when it is used for binge eating disorder exclusively, it can slow down the reoccurrence of binge eating episodes. This is the "first FDA –approved medication to treat binge eating disorder"; however, it is not all sunshine and rainbows (WebMD). Lisdexamfetamine has its share of less desirable side effects. These side effects include, "dry mouth, trouble sleeping, increased heart rate, and a jittery feeling" that is similar to drinking too much coffee (WebMD). These are the milder side effects. The more serious risks to taking Lisdexamfetamine are heart attacks, strokes, and even "psychiatric disturbances" (WebMD). If one is wondering what a psychiatric disturbance is, it is classified as a mental disorder. In other words, it is "a behavioral or mental pattern that causes significant distress or impairment of personal functioning" (Wikipedia). For example, one of these patterns can result in bipolar disorder. As one can see, despite Lisdexamfetamine's benefits, there can be some severe problems that can arise from use, and the problems of binge eating disorder can get worse.

Similar to Lisdexamfetamine, Topiramate (Topamax) was originally used to treat other health problems other than binge eating but has now been adapted as a common treatment for binge eating disorder. Originally, Topiramate was used as an antiseizure drug. While in many cases this drug successfully reduced the number of binge eating episodes, it also brings with it some side effects that are not favorable. These side effects include "memory loss, tingling sensations in fingers and toes, trouble speaking, and sedation" (WebMD). As one can see, medication may help for a while, but if you are not one of the lucky ones that are not affected by the side effects, you open yourself up to a whole new group of problems that you did not have before. Currently, these are the only two drugs commonly given out by physicians to treat the symptoms of binge eating disorder directly; the only other medications are prescribed to treat mental issues that ensue after a binge eating disorder diagnosis has been reached.

Depression, anxiety, social phobia, and obsessive-compulsive disorder are just four of the mental issues that occur when someone has binge eating disorder. Therefore, it is common for doctors to prescribe antidepressants such as fluoxetine (Prozac). This is a very indirect way to treat binge eating disorder because it doesn't exactly affect any of the direct issues that occur. All it will do is help you with those above four mental issues. Another problem is that if you are under the age of eighteen, it is rare that a doctor will prescribe fluoxetine or any mood stabilizer for that matter. Also, antidepressants should never be used without constant monitoring of a therapist. The only reason one should use these is if they are continuing with their self-help process or cognitive behavior therapy treatment. Furthermore, they have some side effects that can be found on their bottle. These side effects include, sleep problems, strange dreams, headache, dizziness, vision changes, tremors or shaking, feeling anxious or nervous, pain, weakness, yawning, tired feeling, upset stomach, loss of appetite, nausea, vomiting, diarrhea, dry mouth, sweating and hot flashes. This route isn't the most desirable, but it is necessary for serious bouts of depression.

There is a third alternative treatment for binge eating disorder, and that is taking a holistic approach. Naturopathic medicine is not practiced at hospitals, personal physicians, and therapists; therefore, it is not covered by insurance companies, and many people believe it to be unproductive. However, this thought process is incorrect and has survived mainly because people do not know much about it. Usually, this idea disappears once someone hears about or works with a naturopath, and they believe that holistic medicine is the missing link in our current health care system. Naturopaths believe in a holistic approach and attempt to use natural remedies whenever they can; they believe in treating the causes as well the disease in its entirety. On top of addressing the causes and the disease, naturopaths also attempt to educate their patients about their illness so that they feel empowered in the future, and the patient can make changes to their lifestyle so that the eating disorder does not return.

Each of these considerations is essential when treating someone with an eating disorder. The holistic approach attacks many aspects on a physiological level. These physiological elements are often what lead to the act of binging and binge eating disorder. Naturopaths will also look at systemic dysfunctions that may be the root or ongoing causes of one's binge eating disorder. Recovering from binge eating disorder is difficult and can have many ups and downs. Having someone like a naturopath, who is understanding and engaged, and wants to look at the issue from multiple directions, can make all the difference in getting better and overcoming binge eating disorder.

As mentioned before, naturopaths like to take the time to educate their patients. Many times people, with and without binge eating disorder, believe that certain foods are healthy for them when in actuality they are not, and in some cases, these foods are creating some of the symptoms they are feeling. In North America, many of the foods are processed, and these processed foods are jam-packed with ingredients to make the food last longer and taste better.

Unfortunately, this is not all these components do, they also make the food addictive and create the cravings that people see in binge eating disorder. If one suffers from binge eating disorder, they often can remember a time and place that they ate something a salty chip, a chocolate bar, or a high sugar beverage that once they started eating it, they could not, or did not want to stop. Of course, this could have a nutritional explanation like the food lacked in a particular nutrient, and that food happened to have it, or there is a blood sugar imbalance, but then there are the times when there is a chemical reaction, and the body makes them not want to stop eating said food. These foods are tough to turn down, so the best possible fix is avoidance. More often than not, this type of food is found in the aisles of grocery stores and the whole foods the ones that are healthy and nutritious are located on the outer edges of the store. Therefore, when one goes to the grocery store try to stick to the periphery and only purchase whole foods. In addition to the aisles of a grocery store, another good thing to avoid would be alcohol, especially if someone is suffering from binge eating disorder. Alcohol tends to manipulate one's judgment. They may know exactly what they should not do such as eating bad foods and binging but alcohol can give them a window to have a cheat day. Once the alcohol is consumed and opens the door to binging or eating unhealthy foods, hypoglycemia can occur. Hypoglycemia is low blood sugar, and when this happens, the low blood sugar will instigate a binge because the body starts craving high sugared food.

Monitoring one's blood pressure is very important for someone who is suffering from binge eating disorder. Sugar in the body regulates cellular function and complications can arise from high and low blood sugar. High blood sugar can lead to things like diabetes, and low blood sugar leads to binging. The diet and nutritional information the naturopath will give one who has binge eating disorder will most likely try to reduce the amount of high glycemic foods like bread and pasta. Another dietary change to be considered is adding meat and things that have healthy fat. These types of foods also have an added advantage; they contain Chromium. Chromium is a mineral that helps regulate blood sugar. Finally, bitters and bitter menu will also be suggested because they lower a person's cravings for sweet foods. They also have the added benefit of improving digestion. Moreover, a naturalist will look at many aspects of the diet—more so than a dietitian or a nutritionist—because they are not just a guide to healthy eating, they are a physician trying to cure a disease.

Dealing with the food a person eats is not the only thing that

Naturopaths do, they also will give you several tests—besides the ones that they will do as an ordinary physician—to determine the causes of the eating disorder as well as attempt to cure it. These tests include cellular micronutrient testing, urinary neurotransmitter analysis, salivary cortisol and hormone testing, and food sensitivity tests. Depending on the individual, each one of these tests may have a place in the recovery of a person suffering from binge eating disorder.

Another cause of binge eating disorder that a Naturopath would be able to determine is a subclinical nutrient deficiency. This means that the body is not producing enough of something which cannot be replenished through diet. Some of the subclinical nutrients include serotonin, glutamate, and norepinephrine. If this is the case, instead of correcting these imbalances with fluoxetine or citalopram like a regular physician, they will attempt to use natural remedies which are much less evasive, but easier on your body.

Along with neurotransmitter dysfunctions and dietary issues, naturopaths would also be able to detect and treat other symptoms like stress, heartburn, gas, and abdominal pain. By doing so, they are staying true to the holistic medicine that they believe in practice. Such things can arise from the eating of large amounts of food in a short period. Finally, hormonal irregularities can result from the crazy sugar intakes during a binge that can lead to mood swings. Adrenal and thyroid disruptions are also a symptom of overeating, and a holistic approach has many more benefits than traditional medicine when it comes to treating these symptoms. Naturopaths and people who practice holistic medicine are well trained to deal with these types of things and often do on a daily basis. Fixing these symptoms with a pill is a short-term fix, holistic medicine aims to fix it for good.

In conclusion, it is obvious that there is no one way to cure binge eating disorder. It is an intricate disease that affects you physically and mentally. For most, the best way to treat the disorder is a combination of the aforementioned treatments and a lot of support from friends, family, and a person's therapist

CHAPTER 5

The Importance of Setting Goals

Setting goals is universal. No matter what it is one is trying to accomplish—whether it be short term or long term—goal setting is essential to success. Whether it be how much or how little sleep to get, whose phone calls to return or not return, how much exercise one will or will not get, how much work one will get done at work or around the house, or how much or what kind of food one eats, goal setting is always involved. Chances are, many people are already familiar and skilled at setting goals; however, how many times does one get to the end of the day feeling happy and relaxed, knowing that they achieved what they set out to do that day?

If one often goes to sleep or wakes up to the sound of their conscience nagging away at them for not accomplishing what they set out to do that day, it is a good indicator that unreasonable or unrealistic goals have been set. Unfortunately, if this becomes a habit, and that conscience is forced to continuously tell them that they did not complete their tasks, then eventually their conscience will start singing another tune; it will start to say that said goal setter will not accomplish what they set out to do and this can become counterproductive. According to Michelle Morand, MA, and founder and director of the CEDRIC center for eating disorders, the answer lies in reasonable goals; "those things that we ask of ourselves that we can actually achieve in a time frame that we set" (Morand). If a goal is reasonable, it should be manageable within the confines of one's everyday routine. It is excellent to want or desire big changes, and it is fine to set lofty goals for oneself when looking at the big picture, but what isn't great is hoping these massive changes occur in a day, a week, a month, and even sometimes a year.

Unreasonable and unrealistic goals do not work in reality, and they lead in only one direction, failure. Failure, "which trigger unmet needs, which triggers the learned helplessness, which triggers anxiety/overwhelm/depression, which triggers procrastination, isolation, and avoidance, and over course binging, purging, restricting (anorexia, bulimia, overeating)" (Morand). As one can see, although setting goals can help deal with their eating disorder, it can also have a converse effect. These kinds of goals tend to fall under the guise of "all-or-nothing" goals (Morand). The ends do not justify the means when it comes to these goals. Anytime someone has to sacrifice all of their energy, time, and emotions into accomplishing a single goal they jeopardize their work, home-life, relationships with others, and their self-care. And, worst of all, if said goal is not accomplished in a timely manner, "you diminish your self-esteem and feel like a failure" (Morand). All of this is done because achieving that goal was thought to be so essential to happiness when in actuality the goal setter's happiness was —slightly if not all together— compromised by the goal itself. Realistically speaking, any goal that places one in a position to neglect themselves, their relationships with others, or their work and home lives is an unreasonable one; and, unreasonable goals put people into a pattern of constant setbacks. This type of goal has one feeling attached to it – and it is failure. Feeling like a failure can almost be worse than being one.

Alright, now that those unreasonable goals and their effects have been covered, how does one get out of this vicious self-deprecating cycle? "For starters, for each key area of your life, career; home; partnership; friendship; family; parent; parent; individual; volunteer; hobbies; et cetera, identify what it is that you would like to see in each of those areas in order to feel truly content and fulfilled like you were living the life you were meant to live" (Morand). After that, then one needs to take a look at where they are now in relationship to said goals. Now that there is a clear picture of the current and desired status, find one step that can be made towards achieving that goal. Once you have that one step, "break that step in half" and then half it again (Morand). Now that one has a quarter of a step towards their goal, they have a reasonable—achievable—goal that can be completed in a short period of time. This first—quarter—step will allow the person some self of accomplishment and momentum that will help build a foundation of further success.

Michelle Morand, in her article, "Setting Reasonable Goals for Eating Disorder Recovery" gives an excellent example of a reasonable goal for someone who is suffering from binge eating disorder:

"Ultimate goal: to never ever use food to cope again and to be a natural weight for my body without effort.

Current state: *eating when I am not hungry at least once a day, most days of the week.*

First step: *I am only going to eat when I am hungry and stop when I am full tomorrow.*

Okay, now let us break that in half: *I am only going to eat when I am hungry and stop when I am full for half of the day.*

And half again: *I am going to have one meal a day where I wait to eat until I am hungry and do my best to stop when I am comfortably full"* (Morand).

Using Morand's example, this person now has a goal that more often than not, they can successfully achieve on a daily basis that does not throw off the rest of their life. This type of goal relieves the pressure to overcome binge eat disorder overnight and lays the groundwork for further successes. Once it becomes a habit to set reasonable goals, success, self-esteem, competency, integrity, and peace of mind will become commonplace, and all of these things will be regular sensations (Morand).

It is important for one to not allow these successes to go to their head. The feeling if accomplishing a goal can lead to believing that it is time for grander heights. It is not—at least not yet anyway. "Typically, you want to give yourself two weeks in the first step, and once you see yourself consistently attaining that goal and feel a sense of confidence with it, you go to the next step" (Morand). When looking at the next step in Morand's example, "I am only going to eat when I am hungry and stop when I am full for half of the day," which essentially means that the person is going to pay attention to their hunger for two out of the three meals (Morand). On the physical level this goal is very straightforward; however, there are two sides to binge eating disorder, and the mental side of this goal is that this person will try to prevent the use of food as a way of coping with certain situations for half of the day. If they can accomplish this goal with consistency, not only will they be binge eating less, they will also be using other tools to combat stress, meaning that they are less likely to overeat in the future.

As one can see, setting—reasonable—short-term goals puts a person in a great position to attain and accomplish their ultimate—long-term—goal. Watching these smaller short-term goals be conquered will create a sense of trust in oneself and their conscience. They will start to actually believe that one day the ultimate goal will actually be able to be achieved. They can imagine themselves at their desired state, rather than only seeing where they are currently.

Finally, when one is first starting out with goal setting—especially when it comes to binge eating disorder—they may want to start a journal. Writing out the first steps in a journal will help assist in identifying what parts of life that need to be changed and visually seeing the first steps needed to be taken towards changing them. "You'll be amazed at the peace and happiness that descends in the first week alone as you see yourself moving forward at a reasonable pace towards the achievement of the life of your dreams" (Morand). When it comes to binge eating disorder, this slow improvement can be what one centers their treatment around.

CHAPTER 6

Positive and Negative Reinforcements and Binge Eating Disorder

Before this chapter goes into how these reinforcements affect someone with binge eating disorder, it is essential to understand what they are. There are four different types of reinforcements that directly impact someone with binge eating disorder, and other eating disorders as well. They are as follows: interpersonal negative reinforcement, interpersonal positive reinforcement, negative social reinforcement, and positive social reinforcement. Each one of these reinforcements effects binge eating disorder differently; some of them are more influential than others.

Interpersonal negative reinforcement is most frequently the source of one's development of binge eating disorder. Interpersonal negative reinforcement is explained as a reaction used to diminish an unwanted internal position. This internal situation can arise from just about anything; their job, their home life, their bank account, and their appearance are all sources of an internal dilemma. In the cases of people who have binge eating disorder, the people suffering use food to eat away these negative feelings; however, this is not logical. The eating—at times—can be the source of this unwanted internal state; thus, this creates a terrible cycle that only leads to failure.

On the other side, there is Intrapersonal positive reinforcement. This type of reinforcement is described as an attempt to cause or strengthen a good feeling inside; for example, happy emotions. In a sense, this could be viewed as rewarding oneself for doing something good. In the case of binge eating disorder, one uses food to continue or sustain this desired internal state. They have often grown up in families that emphasize food and mealtime; thus, they have learned that after doing something right, a good meal should always follow. The problem with this thought process is that—although initially, the person may feel good about eating—the meal is almost inevitably accompanied by negative feelings about themselves.

The third most common reinforcement seen in people suffering from binge eating disorder is negative social reinforcement. Social negative reinforcement is the act of avoiding social interactions or escaping social responsibilities. Nervousness is a frequent companion with this type of reinforcement. When one feels nervous around others or performing specific tasks, they will turn to something that is reassuring, something that they know plenty about. When it comes to people suffering from binge eating that thing is food. To avoid topics at parties that people don't know much about they go in search of people that are surrounding themselves with the food available. If there is food at the party, people will spend more time at the buffet or snack platter than socializing; thus consuming food when in actuality they do not need it or are not hungry. Although this action eliminates the feeling of nervousness, it ends in a much worse result by feeding the binge eating disorder.

Finally, the last reinforcement displayed by those suffering from binge eating disorder is positive social reinforcement. This reinforcement is received by getting attention from others or conveying information to others at a party. This is similar to the previous reinforcement in the sense that people with binge eating disorder search out something reassuring —food— to get through an evening out of the house. Whether this results in someone displaying their ability to cat more than the rest of people at a buffet, or attempting to eat the burger at a restaurant that gets their picture up on the wall, they are all attempts at getting attention from their eating ability.

CHAPTER 7

The Importance of Healthy Food and an Exercise Plan

$\mathbf{A}$ nutritious and healthy diet is a good idea for everyone, not just people with eating disorders; however, it is especially crucial for those suffering from binge eating disorder. During a binge eating episode one loses control of their ability to stop eating; therefore, having healthy, clean, non-processedd foods lying around can at least curb the effects of the episode. Whole foods like vegetables, fruit, eggs, chicken, and beef are processed by the digestive system differently than things like bread, pasta, beans, and cheese. The whole foods go through your system faster and contain many more nutrients that the body needs; thus, it is much more difficult to pack on the pounds. Whereas, bread, pasta, beans, and cheese move through the system slower and can result in the production of fat cells. A nutritious diet is more than just knowing the caloric count of a piece of food.

Although knowing the number of calories one is consuming is a good way to make sure you are not taking too much food in, this knowledge doesn't stop a person from binge eating. To restore and maintain a healthy weight and a healthy relationship with food for those suffering from eating disorders, nutritional education and nutritional therapy should be integrated into the treatment plan.

For this to work, dietitians and nutritionists should have a complete food history. Food history is something that will give a detailed account of your dietary habits. According to Courtney Kent, in her article, "The Necessity of Nutrition in Eating Disorder Treatment," registered dietitians have found that these food histories can actually be more practical than current food intake or laboratory tests when trying to identify nutritional deficiencies or, in the case of binge eating disorder, dietary surpluses (Kent). Once they have discovered where the issues lie in your current diet, a plan can be put in place to correct these deficiencies and surpluses. Fixing these problems in a person will have an array of different benefits. These changes will improve general health, physical recovery, positive mood enhancement; the patient will have a more restful sleep (Kent). Registered dieticians are an imperative part of the treatment process for anorexia, bulimia, and binge eating disorder because they understand many of the psychological symptoms that come along with said disorders symptoms like, co-morbid illness, depression, and boundary illness. The registered dietician can work hand in hand with a therapist all through treatment, as well as provide more structured meal planning as many entering into treatment may have no idea what a healthy meal looks like (Kent).

After a strict meal plan has been set in place and the person suffering from binge eating disorder has stayed true to it, nutritionist, dieticians, or treatment center staff may try to work towards something that is called intuitive eating. Because those suffering from eating disorders not just binge eating have created an ugly connection with food. This relationship needs to be broken, and a new belief system needs to be put in place so that one can once again find joy in nourishing their body. Re-learning how to respond to your body's signals of hunger and fullness can be difficult for one suffering from binge eating because they have programmed themselves to ignore their hunger pains or emotionally overeating past the level of comfort (Kent). This is no longer a practice of psychotherapy; it is called nutritional therapy which differs slightly from the former in the sense that nutritional therapy is mainly focused on food, body image, weight, physical activities, and thought patterns that restricted one from living a full and healthy life (Kent). Binge eating disorder is both an emotional and physical disease so one should always remember that they need more than just therapy, nutritionists are an essential part of the equation. Remember, if one is dealing with an eating disorder it is essential to attempt to find treatment as soon as possible; the longer one waits, the more difficult it is to break away from it.

Nutrition is not the only part of having a healthy and balanced lifestyle, exercise is another integral part of returning to a reasonable weight and fighting against binge eating disorder; however, there are forms of unhealthy activity as well, so it is important to know the difference and exercise in moderation.

Often, binge eaters construct their work out regiments similarly to their eating habits which usually results in an all-or-nothing scenario. People suffering from binge eating disorder tend to try and make up for their episodes all in one go, exercising with a no pain, no gain kind of attitude.

Unfortunately, exercise does not work this way. One needs to work out in moderation and exercise consistently. If one does an extremely difficult work out one day, but then sits around the house and eats the rest of the week, that works out will show no benefits and that person's weight will continue to climb. When working out with the no pain, no gain approach, a person will burn their muscles out in one day and then be too sore to do anything the following two days. As one can see, this will inevitably make the person dislike working out because it causes pain. It will create a psychological resistance do exercise because they will begin to associate it with pain. When this occurs, exercise can eventually be seen as an enemy, something to be endured and not enjoyed.

For those who suffer from eating disorders, this negative relationship with exercise needs to be overcome to improve one's health and their contact with their body. Unfortunately, eating disorders can affect one's mobility and their ability to exercise effectively. Finding a way to exercise healthfully in one's current body is extremely important for the binge eating disorder recovery process. One way to finding this healthy way of exercising is not to view working out as a boot camp, but instead, try to consider working out as not only doable but enjoyable.

It is this change of one's view of exercise that will allow them to feel empowered and even confident in their ability to get better and defeat their binge eating disorder. Often this is tough to do by oneself. It might be a good idea—if the clinic or treatment center does not have something already in place—to hire a personal trainer. They are trained to help people with these types of disorders and should be able to set up a fitness regimen adapted to one's needs. Hopefully, after training with a professional and realizing that, regardless of one's physical situation, exercise is possible and that they want to continue to be healthy even after they finish their sessions with their trainer.

In cases of binge eating disorder, often the person suffering becomes disconnected from their body and they start to tune out what their body tells them. Therefore, exercise becomes more than just a physical test; it is a mental one too. Before working out, one should practice mindfulness and try to get back in touch with the thoughts, emotions, and feelings that they have disregarded for so long. To do this, one needs to forget about the past and not look towards the future, but instead focus on the here and now. This will help them to get in touch with their physical core and be able to feel their bodies. To center oneself, a conscious effort to align the spine and find their balance needs to be done. By doing this, whether they are walking, running, or strength training, the person is concentrated on listening to the body, and their thoughts cannot drift away to something that is not important at that very moment.

Earlier in this chapter, it was mentioned that people are dealing with binge eating disorder approach exercise with an all or nothing approach and how it is ineffective. They need to slow down and stop thinking about the end goal. Usually, when one exercises with the all or nothing approach, they work out at a ten—this is in a one to ten scale, one being the lowest intensity and ten being the highest. Working out at a ten once again tricks one's brain into thinking that exercise is challenging and contributes to the negative relationship they have with exercise. They need to find the middle ground.

Many programs for people with binge eating disorder are attempting to break this negative relationship, so instead of having them exercise at a ten; they will teach them how to do it at around a five. Regardless whether they are doing cardiovascular, strength, or flexibility training, a moderate intensity should be what they are aiming for. Doing so will create confidence in oneself to be able to get through an entire work out as well as leave them finishing their exercise feeling good about themselves and their ability to do whatever it is that they have chosen as their exercise. Once these feelings start to arise in the person suffering from binge eating disorder, they will also begin to believe that their physical goals can and will eventually be met. Because these kind feelings will start to be attached to the thought of exercise, the middle ground method becomes a psychological reinforcement toward exercise adherence, making the person want to go back to the gym, rather than stay at home on the couch. Learning not to dread going to exercise is a very important part of the treatment of binge eating disorder.

Another part of taking the intensity level down in ones work out is that it gives them a chance to modify their exercise to their body's specifications. Binge eating disorder usually leads to weight gain and weight gain can bring with it other problems such as less mobility, shoulder pain, knee pain, and lower back pain. Just because these are issues, does not mean that exercise is impossible; it says that the exercise needs to be modified. One needs to work with their body's restrictions, not against them. Monitoring one's restrictions forces an awareness of their body, something that has been neglected in most who are suffering from binge eating disorder. This recognition will make exercising more comfortable and entirely possible and could lead to the enjoyment of exercise. This will heighten the chances of someone exercising longer and the consistency with which one works out.

Just because the intensity of the workouts has lessened, does not mean that one should lose sight of their goal, losing weight. As this book has mentioned before, goals are supposed to be taken in baby steps. The purpose of losing weight is still there, but it has been chopped up into tinier, more achievable pieces. It is true that lowering the intensity will burn fewer calories, thus taking longer to lose the not so desirable weight. But, this is playing the long game, and instead of focusing on the end goal, it is focusing on a smaller more achievable one like increasing endurance, increasing strength, and increasing flexibility. Therefore, the focus shifted from weight loss to taking care of oneself. This also allows one to keep their expectations realistic and helps build upon their successes rather than being stuck over thinking about their weight. And, this way the person suffering from weight loss can see positive results even if they are not on the scale. Focusing on the numbers on the scale too much can lead one right back to the all or nothing pattern of exercise and—even worse—relapsing into binge eating.

Finally, when it comes to exercise a variety of different activities are a good way to keep things interesting. If one does the same routine over and over again, they will get bored of it. Also, if one does many different activities, they sometimes start to feel like hobbies rather than forced exercises. Here are a few examples of healthy exercises that one might want to explore: dancing, walking, running, canoeing, kayaking, snowshoeing (in the winter), yoga, pilates, basketball, volleyball, and lifting weights. The beautiful part of all these activities is that you can do them alone or in a larger group, and you can either do them inside or outside—minus the snowshoeing. If someone is suffering from binge eating disorder and they are not used to—or do not have much experience with—physical activity, it is a good idea to try a medley of different ones to find out which ones they enjoy, or at least can tolerate doing on a regular basis.

Never try to fit into another person's idea of fitness; one should always attempt to blaze their own trail. That way, one can find what feels right. Feeling good about an exercise approach will help to keep one on track and eventually reach their goal of weight loss. Furthermore, it will assist in making fitness a part of a person's life rather than just a means to an end. In doing so, the negative thoughts about one's body will disappear, and a positive connection will start to form. This is crucial to the recovery and treatment process of those suffering from binge eating disorder.

Another way is to get attention. Binge eaters will impress those around them with their knowledge of food or by even explaining their disease. These actions, because of the attention factor, keep food as an important element of their image and only solidify the binge eating disorder in the individual.

Altogether, positive and negative reinforcements affect each other differently. It is essential for one who is suffering from binge eating disorder to understand their triggers and attempt to stay away from them. Whether it is interpersonal negative reinforcement, interpersonal positive reinforcement, negative social reinforcement, or positive social reinforcement, the result is always the same. The reinforcement furthers the importance of food in said person and, consequently, furthers to control the hold binge eating disorder has on them.

CONCLUSION

Thanks again for taking some the time to download this book!

You should now have a good understanding of binge eating. This knowledge will help you live a happy and healthier lifestyle. Fighting binge eating disorder can be really hard, but it doesn't mean you can't do it.

If you enjoyed this book, please take the time to leave me a review on Amazon. I appreciate your honest feedback, and it really helps me to continue producing high-quality books.

www.ingramcontent.com/pod-product-compliance
Lightning Source LLC
Chambersburg PA
CBHW071240220526

45468CB00002B/932

9781985072879